Burn

Buster

Second Edition 2019

Discover your Red Flags

and what to do about them

Pam Burrows

Dedication

This book is dedicated to my mum who taught me, by example, how to give all your love, and then give some more.

And to Annie, my partner and Director of Everything, without whom lots of wonderful things, including this book, wouldn't have happened.

About the author

Starting her career in child care, mostly because she loved to play, Pam Burrows quickly realised she had a fascination for people; sussing them out, communicating, story-telling and pondering what makes us all tick. She went on to qualify as a social worker but quickly became involved in the training world in the public sector and eventually began training business people internationally in the art of sales and negotiations. So, with a variety of people, environments and skills under her belt, in 1999 she set up her own business to deliver keynote speeches and workshops on the things that make us humans tick.

She is a Master Practitioner in Neurolinguistic Programming (NLP) and is a Fellow of the Professional Speaking Association.

After a number of her own burnout experiences, she offers you this book. Hoping it's short enough to read all the way through and make a positive difference to you and people you know. It's more pleasant to prevent than recover from burnout!

And once you've been there, it's really important to learn how not end up there again.

Alongside one of her customers, Nottingham City Homes, Pam was awarded the European IOSH award for addressing stress in the workplace. She was invited to speak at the UK Health and Safety Executive National Stress Summit as a result.

Pam spends most of her work time delivering programmes to help organisations reduce stress and develop sustainable well-being cultures.

If you'd like to get a little boost from Pam every Monday morning, sign up for her Monday Motivator Message at www.pamburrows.com

She gives energetic and motivating keynote speeches at conferences and her workshops for teams inspire positive change. You can get yourself a boost via her online programmes and a whole host of free feel good resources on her YouTube channel: www.youtube.com/c/pamburrowspeoplebooster

If you want to talk to Pam about the perfect well-being programme for your team or organisation, drop her an email at pam@pamburrows.com

What people say about Pam, Professional Speaker.

"...Pam gives so much more than 'dial-a-speaker'. She fully engaged with us and quickly became a key part of our delivery team" *Taz Foster, Team Leader at Moving Forward.*

"After Pam left, the buzz around the group was about her presentation and it left a good feeling. Even our boring AGM that followed became enlightened, a seriously big thank you!" *John Simmons, Chair of Derbyshire Healthwatch Board.*

"Pam has helped our staff team change how we see challenges, developed strategies for resilience, boosted our positivity and we had a good laugh along the way" *Cat Thornton, Head Teacher.*

"Pam is a breath of fresh air every time she works with our group. She also gives us something useful to make a positive impact back in the workplace, we book her time and time again, there's always something valuable to take away" *Karen Bonser,*

Chair, Nottingham Association of School Business Managers.

"At the HSE National Stress Summit Pam engaged the room and gave everyone useful, practical ideas on tackling work related stress" *Peter Kelly, Senior Psychologist, The Health and Safety Executive.*

"Pam is able to lift my spirits and help my staff build strategies for a stronger mindset" *Justine Drury, Principle, Channeling Positivity.*

"She's a star! She brings energy and insight into every national sales event we book her for" Ian Smith, National Sales Manager.

"I'm very proud" Pam's Mum.

"She's definitely got some Jedi Mind Tricks going on, I only asked her for directions and we've been together ever since" *Pam's partner Annie*

Acknowledgements

Thank you to my Mum, Penny Haslam, Ian Smith, Rebecca Jones, Nigel Risner, Dr Lynda Shaw, Daksha Patel, Rob Brown, Steve Thurlow, other precious friends, customers and colleagues and all the executive level burnout survivors who chose to remain anonymous, for generously sharing your stories with me when I said I was writing this book. I've only included some of their stories here, but all of your experiences informed the content and tone of the book, everything was useful and heart-felt and I am very grateful for your honesty.

And thank you to all the people, close to the edge and over the edge that I have worked with over the years – your stories have fueled my pursuit of solutions to that age-old challenge of not burning out when you care so much you often give more than you actually have.

I hope that we will all remain generous-hearted but achieve the magic balance of keeping something in our own tank too.

Contents

A cold cup of coffee, a missed lunch, a cancelled catch-up with a good friend, an abandoned hobby...what have these things got in common, and even more importantly, do they ring a bell?

In motor-racing, a Red Flag tells drivers to beware of an upcoming hazard, to drive with caution and not to overtake. These things above are the Little Red Flags that help you avoid hazards up ahead such a physical, mental or emotional ill-health and other consequences of doing too much for too long. They might appear to be unconnected, ordinary things, but they suggest the behaviour pattern of someone who is out of balance. Someone who is missing the small, important daily wellbeing habits and thinking they don't matter.

When we don't have enough time or energy for the very things that would help us cope and stay healthy in busy or stressful times, it's a real Red Flag. We have plenty of excuses as to why a skipped a meal or a missed swim doesn't matter. And when those around us start to notice, and to worry, we trot out phrases like: "Stop worrying about me, I'm fine!"

when actually what we mean is "I know I'm not ok, but I can't (don't know how to or scared to) do something about it."

Whether you're reading this because you want to help someone else who is close to the edge, because you've already burnt out yourself, or feel at risk of burning out or you just think stress plays too big a part in your life right now, you might benefit from knowing the answers to the following questions:

How do I know if I might be burning out, what are MY Red Flags?

If it's so damaging, why do I do it?

And how can I stop it happening?

What is Burnout?

There are academic and medical definitions but in simple terms I'm talking about any situation where pressure has caused stress and that stress has affected someone so seriously, they can't carry on. It might be causing a serious health issue or mental or emotional overload. Or all of the above!

Years ago, people talked about it as a nervous breakdown; an overload of the nervous system which then affects mind, body and your ability to get on with whatever you're supposed to be doing.

Burnout can bring on feelings of anxiety, depression, self-doubt, anger and physical illness.

Whatever the definition of burnout, in this book I'm referring your body, mind or spirit saying, "That's it, I can't take any more". There might be a straw that broke the camel's back and a moment of realisation after months or years of build-up, or it might be an extended experience of overwhelm. And although the body, mind and spirit are saying "That's it, I can't take any more!", you might not actually stop even though you have, to all intents and purposes, already gone 'pop'.

Whatever it looks or feels like, burnout does what it says on the tin. There's no fuel left, you're all burnt out.

In over 25 years of helping people in distress in one form or another, I have noticed some reoccurring themes about stress and burnout. I've experienced burnout first hand and I've helped myself, lots of clients, and also my Mum, to find recovery.

There are tell-tale signs that all is not well. It's possible to learn to spot those Red Flag warning signs and build a life full of Burnout Busting habits that create a life of sustainable wellbeing.

'You're heading for burnout when...' Have a look, see what you recognise!

I hope this book gives you some clarity, reassurance and some hope for a healthier, more balanced future.

C is for Compassion. Being 'Kind in your Mind'

1. When you say, "It's ok because I love what I do".

Ah, the curse of the passionate person! Whether you're an employee, an entrepreneur, volunteer or caring for someone you love...how on earth can you take time off from something you enjoy so much?! You might even find that evenings, weekends, holidays, are all just opportunities not for rest but to do more of what you love. There's more than your wellbeing at stake here though. If you really love what you do, you probably want to do your very best at it. Yet when we keep at it full pelt, we lose energy and creativity and ultimately, even though you might kid yourself, you're not giving your best performance.

Real Stories: Loving what you do can mean you mask any feelings of things not being well. Nigel, a speaking colleague of mine, spoke to me about his experience of burnout; a brain aneurysm which appeared to come 'out of the blue'. Or did it? Nigel's in his early 50's, his GP expressed concern at his high blood pressure, so Nigel set to and lost some weight, got fitter and felt much better. He told me "I love what I do, and I don't need much down-time". He felt tired but always put that down to working hard.

Oh, and he wasn't sleeping well. The little red flags were accumulating but it seems if you love what you do, you can excuse away any number of clues that all is not well. His GP was happy about the weight loss but still a little concerned with his blood pressure. Nigel would travel sometimes 3 or more countries in one week and on a particularly packed day in the UK took a £270 motorbike taxi ride in order to get to his third talk of the day on time. "The adrenalin keeps you going" Nigel commented, "and it masks the problems". And then your brain goes pop.

Burnout Buster – Compassion Whether you work for yourself or someone else, you need to behave like you are your own manager. Treat yourself like a particularly valuable employee. Draw up some minimum standards for health and wellbeing. I used to say yes to work in the daytime, evening and weekends. Now, post burnout, I almost never work anything other than weekdays and try to keep some of those free of customer facing work so that I can develop new things and keep up with administration. These are days when I know my adrenalin levels are lower which means I can make a proper audit of how I'm doing. Make yourself take time to do something else, it's healthier and more nourishing for the work you love doing too.

Be kind in your mind, recognise what you need and value that.

2. When you're in pursuit of perfection

Did you know that Arabian carpets are made imperfect on purpose? The idea being that nothing should be perfect except God, so slight imperfections are sewn into the design. Unless you were a fully enlightened being (if there really is such a person) the pursuit of perfection is, in reality, a journey of self-criticism. And I suspect if you were fully enlightened you might realise the futility of pursuing perfection. Like many aspects of human behaviour, it's not all black and white, it's about balance. Of course, we want things to be the best we can make them, but can you ever win? Do you ever get to say "Ah, there it is, well done me!"? Often? Ever?

Real Stories: I have coached several people at director and CEO level who talk about needing to be seen as strong, in control, confident and unflustered in a crisis. That makes sense, unless that's not how you're actually feeling. There needs to be a moment of letting go of the tension and pressure, being real and getting recharged at regular intervals.

One leader suggested that hubris is toxic for an organisation; everyone kidding themselves and others that everything is fine. I once remember a radio interview with a consultant who had been invited to help a commercial organisation with their burn out problem. Staff were staying until 11pm to get work done and the cracks were beginning to show. She interviewed everyone confidentially and one amazing fact came up with every person: they didn't need to stay late but as everyone else was, they didn't want to be seen as not busy enough. The culture of working hard or at least being seen to work hard, and still appear like everything is fine was certainly toxic in that company. The very fact that we now have the word 'presenteeism' in our vocabulary to describe people working for more hours than they are paid for (and still coming in to work when they are ill) speaks volumes. Some organisations have estimated that presenteeism costs them more in the long run due to people simply wearing out.

Burnout Buster - Compassion If you can work out beforehand what would be a 'good enough' result in each situation then you will both know when to stop and when to celebrate success. Stop setting impossible targets and then beating yourself up along the way. You might set a big goal, but you need to notice the little wins along the way and know when to stop pushing. One of my least favourite motivational sayings is 'Never Ever Give Up'. Actually, sometimes giving up is exactly the right thing to do. And then look back and realise just how hard you tried against all odds. If you do your best and work hard, that's good enough.

Be kind in your mind: "Well done me today, I did the best I could and it's good enough".

3. When you have to deserve a break. "I'm not allowed a holiday yet, I haven't done enough"

If you are driven by the need for things to be perfect, to avoid disappointing people, to prove you're good enough, to feel like you've earned your pay or rest time, it's hard to make a holiday happen, after all, there's always something else to do!

Do you struggle to take a rest or a holiday because you have to feel like you've earned it? There's a danger that, a bit like perfectionism, you never quite feel like you've done enough to just switch off. If this sounds like you, start noticing what you ARE achieving rather than what's left to do. There'll always be something else to do and rarely will a huge space appear in your life at the perfect moment in which you can take a holiday – you have to create it.

Burnout Buster - Compassion Trust me, it sounds a good time to book a holiday. Even if it's quite a way off in the diary, get it booked in. If you've just had one, book the next one. And honour it, no cancelling, no taking work with you, now cutting it short. Rest, have fun, switch off, recuperate. It's an order. The alternative is really not worth it in the end.

You can't carry on indefinitely without a break or holiday. Speak kindly to yourself, you're worth it.

4. When you fear of letting others down. Don't be a disappointment!

If you keep pushing yourself to do more than you're able to because you're afraid of letting people down, guess what happens? If your energy, time and enthusiasm are out of balance, you'll end up letting them down more often. You'll find yourself saying yes when you should have said no and then cancelling at the last minute anyway because you just can't fit it all in or you got ill from being overcommitted.

For me this is epitomized by that disappointed voice my Mum uses, using my full name 'Oh...Pamela' to respond to my hair being too short or when I got a speeding ticket. It doesn't matter how old I get, that feeling of having disappointed her is like a stone in my belly.

You could drive yourself crazy trying to be all things to all people and never disappoint them, it really is impossible. A counsellor once told me "You're wearing yourself out trying to help. It's like you're shovelling madly, trying to fill in a bottomless pit and the person whose hole it is stands there watching"

Sometimes you've got to put the shovel down. It's ok to not be a superhero. That way burnout lies.

Real Stories: Ian, a fabulous National Sales Manager, talked to me about his burnout story, one close to my heart as aside from being a great customer, Ian has become a friend. With increasing sales targets in the midst of a declining economy, Ian realised – with the value of hindsight! – that he'd continually blamed himself for the company not hitting targets. Rather than people thinking less of him, he worked even harder, worked longer days and spent more time away from home. He was firefighting for all he was worth but still only standing still in terms of results. His partner could see cracks appearing but her subtle hints that he needed a holiday didn't register as an urgent necessity, even when his boss told him he needed a holiday, the only urgency was to improve sales, and anyway it would take a week to unwind so there was no point taking a break.

Ian remembers "I couldn't have relaxed on holiday anyway so there was no point. You think you're invincible, it's as if just because you got through yesterday means you can do tomorrow. And they were all long days, there was always something to finish off, no matter what time of night it was. Problem solving took over my mind, I was completely occupied by the need to sort everything out, it became more important than eating, sleeping, resting, anything".

Burnout Buster – Compassion Notice what's driving you and check if it's an old tape playing in your head. Is it useful? Is it encouraging? You can choose what goes on in your own head. Make a mental note of the things you know you're good at, your qualities and the characteristics people value about you. Even if you have good intentions, there will be times when we let people down. If you can avoid that, great, but if you can't, do the best you can for plan B and the rest is down to the other person, they have to find a way to reset their expectations.

Make a proper judgement of 'What's the right thing right now' rather than always basing your decisions on your good intentions. You can want to do the kind or helpful thing and still say no. You are still a good person!

Be kind in your mind and remind yourself you're a person with good intentions, even when you're not able to help someone.

5. When it seems you're damned if you do, and damned if you don't

You know you're in a bad place but can't see an acceptable way out? You feel stuck between two evils: knowing you're under too much stress but not being able to work out what to do about it. In some ways it's worse than being oblivious to the problem, at least then you carry on regardless.

Burnout Buster - Compassion Check in with other people, there WILL be another way, another choice if you open yourself up to the possibilities. You might need to let go of the need to be in full control of it all, the need to be right or the need to succeed. You might need to consider changing direction entirely. What is blocking you from finding a solution? As Einstein said, "You can't solve a problem with the same thinking that got you into it". Find someone who can help you take an objective view and see a different way forward.

Let yourself believe there is a way out, you don't deserve to stay stuck in an unhealthy stressful situation.

6. When you're trying to be all things to all people

Like the service sign that says, "Choose two - You can have it GOOD, FAST or CHEAP!"

Are you trying to give all three? Does it feel like spinning plates and that something is always falling off the list? Let's put the service sign into a burnout context, the three choices are:

- Effective

- Overly-Busy

- Healthy

Burnout Buster - Compassion You can't be all three. Certainly not for any length of time. What are you trying to nail? Being too busy, trying to stay effective and wondering why you don't feel healthy? Or are you too busy and trying hard to be healthy too? Something has got to give.

Ease off telling yourself you 'should' be able to do it all and still smile. Listen to your body and mind, what's actually a reasonable way to tackle the situation?

7. When you're mind-reading, imagining what terrible things others think about you

This is a bit like perfection-thinking but potentially more toxic. You're already striving for perfection and then you're imagining the worst possible criticism someone might throw your way. You approach everything you do with the intention of leaving nothing you can be criticised for. It's exhausting and also impossible, we all make mistakes or forget things at some point. And even when the finished job fits our exacting criteria, someone else might still find fault because that's just what they do. If you're striving to do your very best and yet still imagining the negative things someone else might be thinking, you're going to drive yourself crazy and wear yourself out.

Burnout Buster - Compassion The toxicity of mind-reading coming from the fact that you can never win. You will always be able to imagine a negative reaction and set impossible standards that no one else is actually setting you. There's a double whammy at work here: you're placing all your self-esteem into the hands of the outside world, other people's opinions and they're not even real, they're ones you are making negative guesses at.

Here's a crazy thought you might not have considered - People may even think good things about you! You can't live a life that no one will have find fault with but here's the thing, if you always look outside of yourself for the answer to "Am I good enough?" you give away your power.

8. When you are in permanent 'overdrive'

Overdrive *noun*:
'A gear in a motor vehicle providing a gear ratio higher than that of direct drive.'
In engineering terms, overdrive is all about a short burst of extra activity when it's needed, say up a steep hill or over rough ground. Human beings are also capable of this. The trouble is, more and more, we find ourselves in situations where that short burst of extra activity is needed over a longer period than first advertised. It becomes the new normal.

The heightened pace continues, the pressure might even increase, and we try to keep up. We begin to forget the value of rest, we might get irritable or unreasonable with those around us. Then we stop doing the very things that we enjoy, the fun things that would normally help us to rebalance. We're focused only on carrying on and doing more.

Burnout Buster - Acknowledge The most important thing is recognising you're in 'overdrive'; that state of feeling almost permanently switched on. You might feel reluctant to stop completely, stopping might feel like a pulling the emergency cord on a train when all the bags fall off the luggage rack! So, it's important to find a way to take a breath, a short break, or just a change of task to refresh and get a rational look at your workload and your wellbeing strategy. More on creating your own wellbeing strategy later.

Acknowledge what you are achieving. Often, in overdrive, we're focused on what hasn't yet been done, what's not going well and what extra pressures are likely to come along tomorrow. Notice how much you're doing, spot what's going well. This will help you regain some perspective.

9. When you're a fixer. "It's all down to me!", "I may as well do it myself, it's quicker!"

In some industries this is rather grimly referred to as your 'double-decker bus rating' meaning, if you were knocked down by a bus tomorrow, what percentage of your role can be taken on by someone else? Would they know where to find things, how to complete tasks, would they be able to keep things ticking over? If nothing could happen without you, you have a high 'double decker bus rating' and this ramps up your burn out risk.

When you say things like "Well, SOMEONE'S got to do it!", beware of martyrdom. Beware also of picking up tasks because you are the one who sees they need doing and you think no one else will. Beware of doing tasks because you always have, maybe it doesn't always have to be that way. And if it happens too often, thinking it's quicker to do it yourself than show someone else how to do it might feel like a short-term win but in the end it's a long-term loss because nothing changes.

Real Stories: At a time when I was running my own business, I also took on the role of chairing the committee for my local LGBT Pride event. There seemed to be so much to do but everyone on the committee was a volunteer with lives outside too and I got more and more overwhelmed by the task ahead. I'll always remember going in exhaustion and desperation to a coach friend of mine. She instructed me to write down all the upcoming tasks I needed to complete. Then she took the piece of paper and tore it into strips so that there was a job on each separate piece. She handed them to me like a pack of cards and ordered me not to come home from the meeting with any pieces, I was to give away every task to someone else in the committee.

I was reluctant; every year, once the long-planned one day event of Pride was over, we lost most of the committee and had to recruit members, I certainly didn't want to overburden them and have to recruit replacement volunteers right before the event even happened! However, I managed the whole challenge and came away from the meeting without any tasks except to chair the group and make sure everyone did what they were supposed to do. Here's the thing...everyone was happy to take on tasks because they felt more involved, trusted and excited about the day itself. And then someone unprecedented happened and it's the reason why I remember this situation so clearly, so many years later: we kept every member of the committee that year, every single person felt valued and committed to playing a part for another year.

There are situations where you really are the only person that can get a job done. There really are situations where the other people involved won't thank you for giving them something more to do. But sometimes, more times than we might realise, we are doing people a disservice by thinking they won't or can't take on something new. Challenge your own assumptions and test it out, maybe you will be doing them a favour by asking them to help.

Fixing is addictive. If you're a 'let's get on with it' kind of person, you take responsibility, and you can't see a problem without figuring out how to solve it, even when it's not yours to fix. Fixing becomes a habit, it usually leads to a feel-good factor too, everyone wants to feel useful and once it becomes a habit, you don't think before you jump in.

An example: I went to collect my car after it's MOT test and there was a car blocking it in. Instead of bothering to get keys and drive it, the mechanic released the handbrake and pushed it a few feet out of the way. I instinctively moved forward quickly to help push and luckily caught myself before I put my shoulder to the task! Not only was I full of cold and tired, it really wasn't my job and if it was too hard for him, he could just fetch the keys! How many times is it a knee-jerk habit, so we end up right in the middle of attempting to 'fix' before we've even made a conscious decision to help?

Burnout Buster - Acknowledge If your work ethic is all about working hard, being of service, doing a good job you'll find this one quite a challenge. It's not, however, about swinging in the opposite direction, it's about making a conscious decision about whether jumping in to fix this particular thing, this particular time is the best way or not. Sometimes people grow most from sorting their own problems, sometimes people are annoyed by offers of help. Sometimes fixing a problem is a nice idea but you just don't have the time, energy, money or resources at the time. And that's ok!

If your current 'to-do' list would crumble without you, you're carrying multiple weights that no one else could step up and do something has to change before something has to give. Figure out what you could let go of by delegating, sharing the task, paying someone else, or asking yourself if some tasks are even necessary and letting them drop off your list entirely. You could think about swapping a task you find stressful or tedious for something you find easy or interesting with someone who has opposite likes or skills. Passing tasks on to someone else might give them a chance to develop a new skill, feel a sense of purpose or a chance to shine.

Drop the martyr behaviour, there might well be situations when you're the only one who can get the job done but if this becomes your mantra, you'll pick up everything and create your own pressure. Check whether you have different behavior at home compared to work, there might be an attitude you use in one environment that would be useful to cut and paste into the other. Once you feel overwhelmed it can be hard to see the wood for the trees, a little audit on what you don't actually need to do might be a good place to start. Who can you teach or encourage to do some of that stuff? It might be good for them! Less Martyr, More Barter – delegate before it's forced upon you!

Acknowledge how much you're already doing and take your superhero pants off for a bit.

10. When you're on a quest to feel good enough

This sneaks in unannounced, even when you think you are quite a confident person. Oprah Winfrey noted one common denominator of all the guests on her 25-year show; every single guest, everyone from murderer to politician, cancer survivor to Olympian, they all asked the same question as soon as the camera went off:

"Was I ok?". Let me repeat, in 25 years, every single person asked the same question.

With the right circumstances we're all capable of questioning our worth. When that drives us to work ever harder and ignore our health, it's a real problem.

Real Stories: I once coached a sales chap called Daniel. I listened in to one of his sales phone calls with an international client and found I had nothing to teach him about sales skills; he was already exceeding all targets. Still, we had some coaching time left so we had a chat. I could see he was fired up but exhausted, so I asked him about life in general. In a flash, it all came tumbling out. He was ill, working more hours than he was paid for and in danger of losing his relationship because his partner was tired of coming second place to his desire to be the best seller in his team. Daniel was on a mission but, until we talked about it, it was a mission he wasn't even conscious of.

He was driven by the desire to prove himself successful enough to his Dad.

Now then, his Dad had died a few years previously. Because Daniel hadn't consciously noticed this driver, he was ignoring all the red flags that things weren't ok, because he was driven by the stronger, unconscious message of 'I'm not yet good enough'.

We didn't have a long conversation and we were in an open office so it wasn't as deep and meaningful as it might have been. But in those few minutes, Daniel recognised the 'good enough' driver for what it was: a road to burnout. There wouldn't have been a target big enough to scratch that terrible itch, no amount of long days and late nights would bring in enough business to quieten that voice. He realised in that moment that he could recognise his amazing achievements, let go of the driver and get his life back or wait until it all hit the fan and who knows what he might lose. I'd love to tell you what happened next, but I left that office the next day and didn't stay in touch. I can only hope that Daniel made the changes. His boss, short term, might have been miffed that he wasn't over-achieving anymore, but it doesn't take a genius to realise that he couldn't have carried on at that pace. We all need to find a sustainable level, 110% leads to debt.

My Mum grew up believing she was not a valuable person and that you should be grateful for what you got and not expect extra. She grew up to be a caring person and worked in caring professions for decades. Being a caring person made her feel of value, and what a fabulous thing it is. The danger is when your sense of self-esteem is wrapped up in that one aspect, it's hard to press the stop button, to care less, even when you are on your last legs.

The challenge made her more resourceful – forming routines and finding creative ways to manage overwhelm meant she managed to carry on much longer. It's an amazing aspect of resilience BUT it can't go on forever. The important skill to develop, is in knowing when to stop. She describes getting addicted to the routine, feeling like a robot and that the fear of changing the routine being scarier than carrying on while so tired.

At night, after she'd put Dad to bed and was thoroughly exhausted, she often said to herself "No more, I can't do this anymore". And the next morning would wake, anxious about what the day would bring, but just carried on. The problem for Mum was that she felt defensive "No one can take this from me, it's my job" and that needing help meant she had failed. As if she'd be found inadequate, which would mean she was doing it wrong and needed to find another new way of coping. Any alternatives to carrying on, all filled her with dread. Your situation may be very different from this, but I think this mindset can occur in any pressurised situation. My Mum's driver to feel needed and not to feel she'd failed, pushed her beyond healthy limits.

Nigel, my professional speaker colleague, describes his new policy of working less post-burnout: "It killed me to say no to the charity work I would normally have jumped to do". It really illustrates this crazy emotional calculation we do; it kills us emotionally to stop doing something, but it will actually kill us physically, if we keep saying yes to working beyond healthy limits.

Burnout Buster - Acknowledge: Check the evidence, there will be a variety of clues that you are doing ok, or even fabulous, listen and accept compliments, stop undermining your own achievements by responses like "oh that was nothing". And even when you're just chilling out, you're still a worthwhile human being, you have a right to be here. You are enough.

If you recognise that you receive your self-worth from one particular direction, you could choose to stop the imbalance before it gets to a critical point. You need to know who you are without that role, to stop being driven by it, or allowing it to define you, find a way to feel good about yourself, even when you are doing nothing at all.

11. When you compare yourself against other people

You are a unique little flower, my sweet! Comparing yourself against someone else might motivate you to try harder in the short term but is a dangerous game if that's how you measure your worth in the world. And those competitive targets can get mighty addictive, overriding your 'I need to rest now' gauge and leading you to burnout.

Burnout Buster - Acknowledge Notice what you are achieving, set *your own* realistic targets and remember it's all about balance. Is beating that next target more important than your health or relationships? If the answer is yes, then make sure you re-balance as soon as that target is reached.

12. When you're the boss – The Head Teacher, CEO, Manager, Entrepreneur and Parent Problem

Perhaps you were a born leader or perhaps you've ended up there because, well someone had to do it. If you're driven to take up the reins, grab responsibility and make sure things happen, if the amount of responsibility or pressure gets out of balance, it could lead to problems.

If the buck stops with you, the pressure is on to not only be responsible, proactive and strong but to make sure no one sees any cracks or doubts. If you're at the top of the tree, there is an additional isolation and façade of 'everything is fine'. I work with some wonderful groups of head teachers. Once of the groups started up because of suicide rates. There's a danger of feeling utterly overwhelmed by the responsibility, cuts in budgets, increases in targets and the sense of isolation that it's all down to you.

Real Stories: I work regularly with groups of Head Teachers and hear firsthand the stories of holding the whole school together, being the one person who stays calm in a crisis and has faith that the whole school will make it through whatever is the current tough challenge whether it's inspections or more budget cuts. In my confidential conversations with Chief Executives and Directors they often talk about the need to be seen to have it all together and to make sure people feel safe that the organisation is in good hands. That's a lot of extra pressure when all you want to is scream "I'm struggling too!", or "I'm not sure I know what I'm doing!" or even simply "This is so tough right now!"

It's all too easy to tell people to 'be authentic' and 'staff appreciate it when you're honest about your own fears' but there's a limit. It really doesn't inspire confidence if you throw your head on the desk and weep on a daily basis, even if that is how you honestly and authentically feel right now!

Burnout Buster – Acknowledge Opening up and talking about how you feel is crucial. Realising you're not alone is also crucial. You need support from the right places, you need a safe person to be honest with and you need to say 'yes' when the right support is offered. If you're not getting offered the right support, you need to go out and find it. You need to have at least one person you can be honest with when you're struggling, someone who really gets what you are experiencing. But you also need someone who can be constructive about what happens next. There's a danger in just letting off steam and getting back at it without any measures to improve the situation to stop you hitting another wall sooner or later. You need both the 'there-there' and the 'what are you going to do about this?'

13. When you ask, 'How on earth did I get this job!?' - Imposter Syndrome

Real Stories: Since leaving school I had worked in childcare until one day when I was in my twenties, I found myself sitting in a high-backed chair in my own office with my own PA in the next room. I had landed a maternity cover post at the Barnardo's charity head office. I answered only to the CEO and hadn't the foggiest idea how I'd managed to land this position. I was convinced that at any moment someone would come into the room, laugh and ask what on earth I thought I was doing before handing me my bag and pointing to the exit. As it turned out, as it nearly always does in these situations, the people around me saw potential and thought I could do that job. I kept replaying the fact that no one else had gone for the job, that they were desperate to have someone in the role, it was only temporary and all the other reasons why I wouldn't normally have ended up here. Actually, the powers that be had faith in me way before I developed it for myself. I'd taken a leap, and it felt like I'd missed out a few of the usual stepping stones along the way. This is the nature of doing new things, stepping up to the next level. Every day is a steep learning curve for which you have to fully concentrate. There's no cruising through one or two tasks that you know so well you can work through them while you ponder what to have for tea or like driving a familiar route without having to look at the road signs. No, when you're in a new position, even the photocopier is a new adventure set to make you feel incompetent! The trouble was I was focused on all those reasons why I didn't really deserve the job and wasn't noticing the little wins I was achieving every day.

This is Imposter Syndrome and it can hit anyone at any level, even the brightest, most talented people.

All it takes is for the majority of tasks to be new to you and the level of authority to be higher than you'd expected at this stage in your life and boom! you're wondering if they made a mistake and called the wrong person after the interviews. You fear people seeing you as weak, incompetent or stupid, that they might spot the cracks, catch you out, realise you haven't got a clue what you're doing. It plays into our childhood dread of turning up in the wrong exam, having done revision for something else entirely.

Burnout Buster - Acknowledge: Most workplaces have quite stringent processes for recruitment and, first up, you need to get your head around the fact that you made the grade, you passed. And yes, they did check. Then, you need to realise two very important things:

- You are succeeding in lots of small ways every day, notice the little wins not just the "eek! don't know how to do this" new things

- Change means that you are constantly doing things for the first time, so it's expected that you will have a period of time where you don't know how to do some things. It will get better. Give yourself some credit and most of all,

give yourself some time. Change is
also tiring, get more than your usual
amount of sleep, good nutrition,
plenty of water and general
relaxation.

14. When you're convinced, "It's not me, it's them!"

When I'm running a workshop on workplace stress, I
ask people what makes them feel stressed.
Sometimes they'll say that the workload, the
pressure and high expectations (sometimes their
own) are the source of the problem. Some people
say they can cope with all of that, but that their real
problem is other peoples' inadequacies.

Without exception, the frustration towards others
isn't a different problem, it just looks like it is.
They're under pressure and just about managing.
Add to this the way they perceive other people and
boom, there's the stress. They might not see it
straight away, but once they start to feel calmer and
clearer, they can see that getting angry with other
people is a sign that all is not well. Additionally,
getting frustrated at other people's behaviour
increases their own stress. And eventually they
understand that their frustrations were a Red Flag in

themselves, a signal of stress, rather than other people being the cause of it.

Which suggests we could all do with a little self-analysis. If you're irritable, tired, under pressure, it might seem like everyone is stupid, taking too long, expects too much or too little, if it feels like people aren't helping, (in fact, they're making it worse) it suggests there's something else going on. Your stress symptoms or Red Flags might manifest as road rage, pavement rage, photocopier rage, computer rage, (you can see where this is going), anything-rage! You really can get frustrated with anything if you're already in a heightened state of stress. It's not possible (trust me) that everyone and everything is out to frustrate you. That mindset tells you the problem is your own stressed perspective. You can get stuck in blaming everyone and everything else or you can take a deep breath and ask yourself, "What do I need right now?"

Burnout Buster - Acknowledge: Noticing that you're mad with everyone is the major breakthrough here. To acknowledge that you're coping with too much and that you're in 'blaming everyone else' mode is the first part and then, *without turning the blame on yourself*, let it go. Make plans to release the tension and work out how you're going to slow it down, take some time out and see the good things, not the irritating ones. If you're in a constant rush, people appearing slow is going to irritate you. You could reframe that to 'they're doing me a favour, helping me take a moment to travel with a smile'. Maybe you need a talking therapy session, a short break, some sport or a proper holiday. At the very least you need to work out what actually is the real problem and then set about solving it, rather than feeling frustrated at anything and everything. Acknowledge what you need and make it happen.

15. **When you're kidding yourself and avoiding reality.**

"Hi, how are you?"

"I'm fine, thanks"

Is this the most told lie of all time?

You might kid other people that you're fine for all kinds of reasons, some of them valid like reassuring a child that they're safe or not letting your boss lose faith in you. And then there's the real problem; when you're not just kidding everyone else but you're kidding yourself.

"It's ok, it's just temporary, it'll all calm down soon".

Really? Is that true? It's all well and good to have a short burst of extra effort - so long as you have the reserves to pull out all the stops for a short time - and just so long as it really will only be a short time. Will it actually calm down soon? How long have you been saying that for? Has this frantic overdrive actually become your new normal?

When an unusual amount of pressure comes your way, you might be able to manage the situation for a short time. If it isn't unusual or temporary then the additional energy required to sustain the extra load starts to cause problems, it leads to burnout.

The Swan Phenomenon - the swan glides effortlessly, gracefully across the lake. Meanwhile, under the water, its feet are flapping madly.

If you're feeling stressed but have to appear like you've totally got it all together at an important meeting or in front of your child's teacher or for a job interview, making like a swan is a fabulous plan. The problem comes when you're 'doing the swan' all of the time. Everyone (unless they know you exceedingly well) will be fooled and no one is able to help or support you because they don't know there's a problem. You have to keep saying yes because there's no obvious reason not to and you have to keep up an exhausting pretense that everything is: "Fine!!! Yes, I'm absolutely fine!!!"

It's a triply tiring situation with the original overload and then the additional pressure of pretending, there's no opportunity to take a break, and you have to keep on pretending. I'm tired just writing about it!

Burnout Buster - Reality: I'm not going to be subtle here. **Stop it. Just stop it.** There is no way to win this long term. Yes, it can be useful, maybe essential in some circumstances to be a swan in the short term.

If you carry on, there is no room for recovery and the problem will only get worse. Stop kidding yourself that it will all calm down soon and you'll magically bounce back. If you don't plan some recovery time, life will just continue to send you challenges and you'll get more and more worn out. If people who care about you keep asking if you're ok and you hear yourself repeatedly saying "I'm fine!" when you're not, take notice. Then you can start to say, "It's hard at the moment but I'm taking a break on ...". Have a plan, stick to your plan. Put something back in the bank. One thing is for sure, the longer you run on empty, the longer it takes to recover.

Be realistic about how much you can handle and how long for. Stop pretending and get strategic about when this 'temporary busy period' will actually end and what needs to be in place, or to change, if it continues.

16. When you're expecting too much of yourself

If you regularly set yourself, say, ten things to do in a day and you only achieve five of them, you could safely say you're expecting too much of yourself. The double whammy comes when, at the end of the day, you only focus on the five you didn't do and beat yourself up for not managing to achieve more. Not only do you end the day missing out on a feeling of satisfaction, you risk feeling overwhelmed by what you need to catch up on tomorrow. You also miss the opportunity to build your perception of your own strengths; when we notice what we *have* achieved, we feel more capable and resilient the next time we're put to the test.

Burnout Buster - Reality: Be realistic about what you set yourself to achieve. Placing things in your diary on the day you're going to do them might help in seeing what will fit and what's beyond humanly possible. Celebrate what you get done, even (especially) the little things and the things you take for granted because they are familiar and easy for you. Acknowledging your skills and achievements will help you feel more resourceful right when you need it.

17. When stopping isn't an option and time off seems weird.

Have you ever had a day off when relaxing feels so weird, you find things to do? Ah, lovely a free Sunday to sit about in the garden, but then you spot the grass needs cutting or you're off to the DIY store to buy a new shed? Maybe you're the kind of person who chooses an activity holiday rather than a lounging about one.

Here's the news. Stopping is always an option. You might not feel like you can stop voluntarily but you can sure stop if it's forced upon you. At some point you're going to come to a stop, and I think you'd rather stop while all your faculties are intact than stopping because you went pop, physically or mentally.

The very fact that you're feeling a real resistance to the idea of stopping suggests you've gone beyond rational and into overdrive.

Feeling like stopping isn't an option might encourage you to find endless 'quick fixes' like caffeine, fast food, sugar products or other fast energy that ultimately will make you more tired, and unwell.

If I had a pound for every person, I've met who was close to burnout and then had an 'accident' resulting in a broken bone or some other health problem that meant that now they really had to stop, well, I'd be able to buy you lunch. A very nice lunch. And maybe even an overnight stay.

Addiction to busy is a real thing. If you feel weird when you stop, it's possible you've developed an addiction to busy. All the busyness, the strain and stress seem to have become a habit. Familiar and addictive in that doing anything other than your to-do list makes you feel uneasy, maybe even guilty. If this is how you feel, you're already a way down the line to burnout or, if this is how you have always felt, you have a greater risk of reaching burnout at some point.

Burnout Buster - Reality: It's ok to enjoy being busy. It's ok to fill your leisure time with things to do so long as they're not work things. If you prefer activity to complete rest, you just need to make sure you're doing something different to work and something that you enjoy. It sets off different chemicals in the body and uses different brain functions so that you feel recharged. Make a plan that includes fun things to do and maybe you could practice having some downtime too.

If busy feels like a permanent state for you, you might need to consider some kind of coaching to help you develop a healthier, more sustainable was of approaching work and life in general. If it's a temporary state or been going on for some time, plan some fun stuff in your free time that still feels you're doing something, it's hard to go from 100 miles an hour to zero. Try something active but relaxing like sport, dancing, family games, a hobby or a small adventure. Just to be thinking about something else other than the thing you've been overworking on will refresh your body and mind.

Don't wait for nature to take its course and force you to stop, you deserve rest and balance in your life. If stopping right now doesn't seem like an option, then when? If it's a big project that can't stop, how can you plan in small breaks or at least some healthy lunches or short walks? How can you keep yourself going, in a healthy way? Make a plan. Make it full of kindness, nourishment and long-term health.

18. When you're saying yes to everything. Over-promising and under-delivering

Are you finding that despite your best intentions, you can't keep your promises? It may well be your 'best intentions' that are the problem. Sometimes it's just not humanly possible to do everything you have set yourself.

I have a new rule which is when someone asks me to help or join in with something, I no longer allow myself to say yes right away – even if I'm really sure it's a good idea. There is a difference between a good idea and a good idea that you actually have the time, focus and energy for. I used to have a knee-jerk "yes!" reaction to nearly everything. I now take some time to consider if I really do have the time and energy and guess what? Some of those ideas turn out to not be so good after all!

Burnout Buster - Reality: What resources (time, money, energy, motivation, interest) have you got in reality? You can seriously damage your reputation with both work and friends by not being able to keep your promises when it turns out you can't follow it through. Operating more strategically will get you more credibility. For instance, saying you need to check first and then coming back with a 'no, sorry' is so much easier than saying 'yes' immediately and then having to let them down later. If you need to say no, it's rarely the catastrophe you might imagine. Especially if you're clear about why you're declining. I recently said no to a piece of work because the exchange wasn't viable, the energy it would take versus what I would get out of it didn't add up. Another job soon came in, one that made me feel more valued and would be a fair exchange. You do get to just say no sometimes and the sky doesn't fall in. And it's important to notice, if you say yes to everything, what are you, by default, saying no to? Health? Calm? Quality?

19. When you give 110%. (hint: it doesn't add up!)

If you pride yourself on 'going the extra mile' or if you're known for giving 110%, that sounds like a good thing, right?

Let's have a think about where the extra mile or that extra 10% comes from. If each day you set out with a certain level of energy and enthusiasm, but you then use up more than you've got, you can quickly see this adds up to some mighty debt. Some people only talk about giving 110%, and it's all flannel. If you actually do give 110% you could be on the way to burnout. If it was a bank account, you'd be racking up some interest and some charges on your overdraft.

Overdrive = overdraft!

Do you overestimate your energy levels and underestimate how much you're committed to? Do you dash about in a reactive way when there might be a smarter way to get the task done?

If energy was a tangible, measurable thing, we'd know when the pot was almost empty. However, we carry on giving it away until it's too late, we're already beyond exhausted. We need to have a conscious awareness of what energy we have and what we're saying yes to. And to see if the numbers add up!

Real Stories: Some life changes come about slowly with a growing realization. For Rob Brown, author and professional speaker, his life changed with a sudden and serious health issue that wasn't burnout related but nevertheless resulted in a huge shift in the way he works. His brain injury and resulting eyesight problems now means that he is unable to drive. Train journeys can mean a really early start and long journey times, so he's connected with local retirees who are happy to drive him for a reasonable fee. What a companionable way to travel! One of Rob's major discoveries was that once we get over our reluctance to ask for help, so many people are really pleased to step forward. "Be specific about what you'd like them to help with, it makes a huge difference".

Rob now works as close to home as possible and rarely accepts work overseas. His business model allows him to connect with people by phone and video calls for which in the past he might have driven up and down the country. It's about getting smart, challenging whether it can be done another way, a solution that uses less energy but still gets great results.

There's a big difference between the intention to do something and the resources to do it. If a friend with a new baby is going crazy from sleep exhaustion and asks you for help, you may well have a kneejerk reaction to say yes because it's the right thing to do. Your desire to be a helpful, caring friend is separate from whether you have the capacity to help. Yes, of course, if a friend is in desperate need you might go over and babysit even if you were totally exhausted yourself, there's that 'pulling out all the stops' things again. The point is to be aware of the decision you're making and to know how and when you are going to get the rest that you need as soon as possible afterwards.

Burnout Buster - Reality: Make an assessment at the start of your day: How are you feeling? What kind of activity would suit your mood, energy level and focus today? What kind of schedule will nourish and sustain you in the light of those answers? Pay particular attention on the days when you really have to do something but don't really have the energy for it. How will you recoup that energy? How will you fuel yourself for the day and keep yourself as balanced as possible? When is the first opportunity to take some recharging time? Then make a pledge to make sure that plan actually happens. It might be as simple as a hot bath after a busy day, be careful you don't end up too tired for the recovery part of your day. Give 100% each day by all means, but make it 100% only of what you, in reality, have in your tank that day.

20. When your diary is completely crammed

Is your diary back-to-back full, so that any emergency or unexpected occurrences really cause problems?

What does your schedule look like? Are there any gaps? And even if there are some gaps in between the booked in appointments, are there 6 million things you intend to do in those gaps that aren't written in the diary? How about the preparation before each meeting and the things you'll need to do to follow up afterwards, are they in your diary too?

How will you make those things happen if there are no spaces? Can you see how we get overwhelmed, beat ourselves up for not getting everything done, when we've almost set it up to fail?

Burnout Buster - Reality: Organise your schedule in a realistic way. Think about what you need get to get done and diary time for it. Be realistic about how long things will take. Diary time for all the things you have in your head that need to be done that you don't normally account for. These are often the things that create overwhelm or a sense of under-performing because they haven't been factored in.

Yes, this might mean you have to say 'no' to some things, but guess what, those things would have fell off your list anyway, you're just allocating time and attention in a more planned way.

Create some Sanity Spaces. Make yourself an appointment with sanity, could anything be more important than keeping your head? I sometimes write this in as 'QTFM', it looks like an impressive kind of meeting and actually stands for Quality Time For Me. This might be a slow lunch, a walk, some time to read or take a long bath, just so long as it's not work or what someone else needs. It's not a luxury, it's refueling that tank.

There's something to be said for planning other gaps in your diary too. Not just for 'you time' but because there will always be unexpected things that come up like you, a family member or pet taking ill, a car issue, a delay in the completion of a project, a pigeon in the chimney, running out of ink or some other unexpected task. If your diary is full, there's no room for emergencies and you're likely to experience overwhelm. Just like money; if you always spend everything you have (or even more!) and then the car needs a new engine or the washing machine breaks, you've got a real crisis. If you've put some money aside for emergencies, it's not quite the crisis it would have been, and you can take up the slack.

21. When people say to you, "But you're always the strong one!"

If you're known for your resilience, your drive to succeed, people will assume you have great resilience. If people know you as a bit of a go-getter, someone they admire for having the courage to go for a big, shiny job or a crazy adventure, it can be harder to step down from the pedestal. If you've always been strong then start to struggle, it's hard to spot, hard to admit and even harder to make the changes, after all, you have the habit of always pushing yourself, how on earth do you take your foot off the pedal but still feel like 'you'?

Real Stories: Penny was doing a great job of presenting the business news on BBC television. She was getting up crazy early, travelling loads and struggling with a number of life crises that had all kicked off at the same time. She was known as a strong woman, a fighter, someone resilient and resourceful so it made it all the harder to say, "I'm not ok, I have to stop". Acknowledging her burnout was the first hurdle, then making the decision to leave a dream job was the second. Sometimes you just have to go with what's right for you, even though it's not what everyone else wants or expects!

For a few years I travelled internationally delivering training courses for a world-renowned research company and people were always excited to ask me where I was off to next. It sounded glamorous and interesting but increasingly I was homesick, lonely and very tired of it all. Any role or even personal relationship, which gives you kudos and which seems to have more pros than cons, can be hard to give up, not because of ego so much as the fact that you and other people can find so many good reasons to keep trying!

Burnout Buster - Reality: It's time for a change. It might have been the perfect role, relationship, business or project when you took it on but now it's killing you. Figuratively or literally. Separate out your desire for success, excitement or challenge with your self-worth; you are a valuable human being even when you're not doing anything at all. Have a long hard look at what you really want and what is good for you, body and soul, not just the title, the travel, the kudos or the pay packet. Would you rather be well and happy?

22. When you have 'brain fog'

If your head is full to capacity and feels like a crazy traffic jam, how can you refocus, plan, and organise? First stop trying to muddle through and take steps to clear the fog. There is a need to get practical with the things you have on your to-do list and also to sort out how it's making you feel.

Burnout Buster - Reality: Get some help to properly assess what you have to do and see what's urgent, what's important and the best way to go about getting it done and still stay sane. Once you have clarity about what needs to be done, what was driving you crazy but didn't actually need to be done and you have a plan about who is going to do what, then you've basically cleared your desk.

Now, very importantly you need to clear your mind. It may help now you have a clear plan but don't underestimate the effect the overwhelm had on you. It's important you don't just crack on with the new plan and find yourself back in the same place x months or even weeks later.

Take some time doing a completely different activity, preferably moving outside.

Learn from the brain fog, it's a really obvious red flag that all is not well. What are you going to do differently to keep things in balance?

23. When you dismiss the concerns of other people (who see your energy dipping)

Every single one of the people I interviewed about their burnout experience remembers someone voicing concern about them. And every single one remembers batting off those concerns and carrying on regardless. Talk about red flags! The clues were there!

How do you feel when people close to you say you're working too hard, not taking enough rest or taking on more than your fair share? If you get frustrated, passing it off as interfering, over-worrying, doubting your capabilities, criticism, jealousy, their own lack of stamina or a lack of understanding of the pressures and importance of what you're doing, there's a chance you've tipped over into a dangerous place. If their worries are really not valid, then why does it bug you so much?

Real Stories: One of the things my Mum recognised post-burnout, was that while she was caring for my Dad at home, with all the issues that came with his Alzheimer's, she didn't listen to the people around her, the people who could see what was happening and were concerned for her wellbeing. Her focus was solely on what her husband needed, on the next thing that had to be done, remaining alert to his safety literally 24/7. Everyone else could see the problem but she couldn't see beyond her next task. She heard us all saying how worried we were but her commitment to caring for my Dad meant she couldn't see any alternative but to carry on. Even when she fell and twisted her ankle, she found a solution - getting around on hands and knees and later with a motorized scooter in the house - rather than solving the root problem; overwhelm and exhaustion.

Burnout Buster - Energy: After the stress subsides or you burn out completely will you look back and wish you'd slowed down earlier, saying "I didn't listen to advice, I was stuck in a hamster wheel"?

Not listening or understanding fully what people's concerns are, not checking with yourself to see what they can see could result in you missing a really important message, and further problems. Disproportionate reactions to small irritations might be a good flag to spot. You might have some communication or some relationship issues to sort too but maybe it's more about your behaviour. Don't shoot the messenger, have some time-out to think, ask the opinion of someone you trust or someone unconnected with the situation so you know they have a no agenda when they tell you if they see criticism or concern. Your worst 'critic' could be your saviour in disguise.

24. When you say, "It's my vocation!" (So there's no time off allowed)

Beyond loving what you do comes an almost martyr-like commitment to the cause. If no one ever felt like this we'd be in a sorry state. It's essential that there are people in our world who get fanatical about doing the right thing. What's counterproductive though is when you don't know where to draw the line, take stock, take a break, see the bigger picture.

Real Stories: My Mum rarely took time off and if my Dad went to a day care centre, she'd spend the time doing all the jobs around the house that she couldn't do with him there. It was so hard to get her to slow down and rest because she always had a really valid reason for carrying on; the jobs needed doing and Dad needed to be cared for. And the crunch: they married for better, for worse, in sickness and in health and it was her job to look after him. She says that her recovery from complete burnout took (is taking) so much longer because she went on far too long after those first signs. It's understandable, even laudable, to follow your passion and keep your commitment to a goal or person. When that overrides your ability to function, it's madness and unsustainable.

Burnout Buster - Energy: If you're really passionate about what you do or who you serve, know that in order to do the best you possibly can you need perspective and to know where you can get support or share the load. As they say on aircraft, you need to put you own oxygen mask on first if you're going to be any use helping anyone else.

25. When it feels like you've pressed the destruct button - Self-sabotage

Sometimes we actually realise you're at breaking point but don't do anything to remedy the situation. Almost like we're letting the truck career down the hill and we're just waiting for the crash.

People admit to me that they seem to be sabotaging themselves. I think it's not so much sabotage really, as being clueless about what they could do the improve the situation coupled with ineffective quick fixes that are making the problem worse. For instance, if you're so busy that you've become completely wired, you might use alcohol to switch off so that you can get to sleep. But then the alcohol disturbs your sleep in the middle of the night and you wake tired. So then you use caffeine to get through the day and end up wired...you can see where this is going.

It also might be the 'addiction to busy' that is at play here; you keep taking on more and more because slowing down or stopping would now just seem weird and maybe even scary. You may also be addicted to the rush of adrenaline and other stress hormones that make it difficult to wind down or take a day off, because you're permanently in full-alert mode.

Burnout Buster - Energy: The best way to handle self-sabotage is to start small. What are the very simple, practical, healthy things you can start to put back in? This will begin to tackle those stress hormones at source.

What's your best way to get a – natural – good nights sleep? What are the nutritious foods and drinks that will help you manage your energy levels? What short but pleasurable activities give you a sense of relaxation or fun? Rebalance your hormones by internal nutrition and external fun.

And of course, longer term, what needs to change? You don't have to wait for the complete crash to make the change.

You can choose to make this right again.

You want some sanity and some energy to put into the new, better way of doing things. Ask yourself, what are you avoiding and what will help you make the positive change you really want to make. Did you ever have a bad cold and have to cancel going to a party that you didn't want to go to anyway? I suspect sometimes we want to 'hit the wall' so we can blame the breakdown for the change. Maybe you could just make the change anyway.

26. When you never quite seem to be 'in the moment'

You're worrying about what happened before, panicking about what still needs to be done and can't quite concentrate on what needs to be done right now. Have you experienced this feeling when you've got lots to do, you finally get down to concentrating on one of the most important jobs but still have that feeling you should be doing one of the other things? You're trying to focus but your mind is off into the future, wondering what you should do next.

Being too busy and experiencing stress can lead to the least healthy form of time-travel, the habit of never quite being in the moment but worrying about what happened yesterday or what's going to happen tomorrow.

Burnout Buster - Energy: Start with some long, slow breaths to calm your heart-rate down. Sit still. Full-on mindfulness (being in the moment) is a mediation practice but you can apply mindfulness to anything and everything you do. It's about bringing your awareness to what is happening right now. In this example of doing one job and worrying about the others, a mindful approach would be to say to yourself "This is what I'm doing right now, everything else will get done in good time" and to give the current task your full attention. Notice the progress you're making and if your mind wanders again don't beat yourself up, bring yourself back gently and kindly to what you're doing right now.

27. When you're living in (not very blissful) ignorance or 'La la land'

There are some warning signs which you either ignore, don't see or don't act on.

If you know that when you start to get clumsy it's a sign that you're too busy, too tired, out of balance or whatever, that's one thing. Ignoring it is quite another. This LRF, Little Red Flag, will just get bigger until you can't ignore it any more.

A bit of clumsiness ignored, might build into something getting broken or maybe an injury. It's hilarious when a child doesn't want to hear you telling them to go to bed, sticking their fingers in their ears and singing "la la la la la ..." but ignoring the signs of impending burnout could have serious consequences.

Burnout Buster - Energy: Take note of your LRFs and make sure you take action to rebalance. You could have a short list of things you know work for you like an early might, a long bath, a chat with a friend or therapist, booking a day off or getting back to eating properly.

28. When everything else matters more than what you need

When we're too busy, it's easy to lose focus on what really matters. Other people's priorities, traumas and concerns can override our own needs. If you work in an emergency service it's even easier to say "ah well, you can't let people down in a crisis". But here's the thing, we can convince ourselves that anything is a crisis, even when the work is paper based not people, we can get engulfed in deadlines and pressure to perform. But whether it's life and death or an end of year report, you can't help anyone if you go 'pop'.

Does your eating pattern, types of food, hydration and other essentials seem as important as getting the next task finished? Neglecting your basic needs

Real Stories: This is something Ian talks about, he stopped eating well, drank more alcohol and always put getting the job done ahead of what his mind or body needed. Ian also suggested that although most

50-year olds are encouraged to have a health check, an MOT, that this should also include a mental health check. You take your car to a professional and make sure it's safe and in working order, we need to do that for our body and mind, especially if we're in any kind of a pressurized situation. If the brakes don't work or the wheels fall off, that's when you know about it!

One of the few people I've spoken to who consistently manages pressure well is an ex colleague of mine, Steve Thurlow. He was a director of the international training company I worked for and though his story deserves a book of its own, here's a snippet. Steve began our chat by telling me "I don't do stress" and perhaps there is something about our characters that makes a difference in that regard. He talks about being self-reliant and relaxed as a child and not especially driven, bordering on lazy (his words!) But key to Steve's lifestyle now was losing his wife suddenly at a young age. He was alone with three young children which meant developing some resilience right off the bat. Steve says life is all about how you tackle a problem, not the problem itself and his motto is that you either sort it or suck it up. When I worked with Steve he was always the out of the leadership team that took time to chat and really listen. He has the kind of open heart that you'd think could lead to too much giving and overload. But he's also canny, he tells me the secret of a good life: "To be lucky enough to have an opportunity, to be clever enough to spot it and brave enough to take it".

Steve is now living out on the coast and walks his dog on the beach. One of many people I've talked to for whom walking the dog brings them so many positive benefits.

Losing his wife gave Steve a life-long perspective on what really matters. He's not a guy to read his emails whilst on holiday.

Burnout Buster - Energy: This is a no-brainer and yet we ignore it so often: eat natural, nutritious food, drink plenty of water, plan ahead so you know you will always have the right fuel for what you need to do, maybe batch cook meals so you'll have something good to eat when you get back too tired to bother. Take packed lunches full of nutrition rather than relying on what will be available when you're out and about. Look after your mental health too and consider having someone that you regularly check in with, whether that's a professional coach or a trusted friend, make sure they can see how you are, and that you heed their observations. Who cares about your physical wellbeing that you can trust to be honest with you? See them as your temperature gauge and check in every now and again to see if you have your priorities right, or sit down yourself and write a journal, read it back imagining it was written by someone you care about. If it sounds like a list of excuses for over work, be honest with yourself and re-set your priorities for good health and a balanced life.

29. When you cancel your favourite things. Pleasure is cancelled for the duration

This is a big red flag - when you've stopped doing the things you really enjoy because you're exhausted or because it feels you could use the time to catch up on everything. But we never do completely catch up once and for all on everything we set ourselves, do we? GPs look out for this particular red flag when diagnosing depression; the very things that make you feel better are the things you cut out when times get rough.

Burnout Buster - Energy: Well, no rocket science here. Get those good things back in the diary. Pronto. And no excuses. No "Oh I want to go back to Zumba but Claire's not going anymore". No "I'd love to go to the theatre but we can't afford it". Go to Zumba on your own. Go to the more affordable local amateur productions. Find a way to do the things that make you feel good. Anything is better than the same blank evening or weekend, over and over, thinking you're relaxing and recharging when all you're doing is vegetating. I have noticed that I might feel too tired to go to my fitness class, I go anyway and after all the games, the laughter, the exercise, instead of tired, I feel more energised.

Focus not on the effort it takes to get there but focus instead on the feeling you'll have afterwards and why it's worth it. Make some memories, make your soul sing, that is what recharges you.

30. When you're in Overdrive and creating an Overdraft – The Consequences

Running on reserve, getting into energy debt is a one-way street. Once you rack up time and energy debt you end up with an overdraft. How do you pay the interest?

If you're noticing recurring illness, (particularly if linked to low immune system) mood changes, mental illness, physical injuries through imbalance, irritability, forgetfulness, problems with communication, understanding and relationships. Aches, pains, headaches, colds, flu, back pain, digestive, sexual problems, heart racing, teeth grinding, skin, eyes, as if your immune system just seems totally conked out, you're paying interest on energy debt.

Real Stories: There's an additional problem if you have a role (paid or unpaid) that generates adrenalin. This can prevent you from accurately assessing what energy you have or haven't got. As a professional speaker I know there's an amount of adrenalin involved. There's the excitement of getting on stage and often a double whammy when you come off stage to a queue of people who want to ask questions, book you for another conference or just to tell you how you have helped them. All the while, adrenalin makes you feel like you can take on the world. I imagine there are some Class A drugs that can give you a similar artificial sense of energy; you take the drug and feel completely energized and positive, you meet, greet and perform your best ever. And then at some point comes the inevitable withdrawal. I often refer to it like someone suddenly took my batteries out! The tiredness hits you and you realise you've done more than you actually had the energy for. After a three-day conference with my professional speaking peers at which I'd delivered a 15-minute workshop 4 times back to back with one minute in between, performed in the stand-up comedy competition and basically talked, listened and networked for between 12 and 18 hours a day for 3 days I was understandably exhausted. But it didn't hit me straight away because I was so high on the excitement, the fun and the adrenalin. I got a really bad cold and cough after that and then came shingles. There is no mystery here!

Rob Brown's faith and his church community has played a big part not only in his recovery but in enhancing the richness in his life. He shared this with me: "When God has a message about your life he'll whisper in your ear. If you ignore it he'll speak up and if you continue to ignore it, he'll start to shout. If you still ignore him, he'll knock you off your bike".

I love that, it really rings true in burnout! If we notice and heed those early Little Red Flags, we prevent the bigger ones coming to get us!

Burnout Buster - Energy: Return to the very basics. What recharges your batteries? You can address any number of your overdraft symptoms but then how will you prevent yourself ending up here again? What needs to change? You are a precious soul who deserves to feel well and enjoy life. What is the right thing, right now that could refill your tank?

You know the phrase 'running on fumes'? When there is so little fuel in the tank the engine must be running on the petrol fumes. You're a strong, resourceful person who can 'go the extra mile' and 'pull out all the stops' but you've done that repeatedly until your reserve tank is empty, you've moved into energy debt.

Keep this knowledge in mind – that adrenalin is only temporary energy and you'll come down on the other side. Plan for downtime immediately after the event. Know what helps you to re-ground and regain balance in energy, mood, eating, sleeping and enjoying yourself.

31. When you can't sleep

How are you sleeping? It's such a common stress indicator and it's no wonder; if your mind thinks it's under some kind of risk, whether it's real or imagined, you'll be stuck on high alert and find it hard to switch off. You might struggle to get to sleep or fall asleep easily but then wake and off your brain goes again.

Burnout Buster - Energy: There are many remedies for sleep; a good relaxing routine beforehand, long Epsom salt baths (the salts get the tension out), the right food, herbal remedies, avoid alcohol, avoid close-up device screens two hours before bed, reduce your caffeine intake, get your room to the right temperature, pillow and bedding, relaxation audios (find mine on YouTube) but actually, if you're still doing all those crazy over-working burnout behaviours, your sleep will still be affected. Treat the cause as well as the symptom and work out what you're worrying about.

32. When you lose your creativity or the quality of what you do

When you're too busy and too stressed, a key thing that disappears is the time to think things through or get creative. You rush through tasks, rush through the day, rush through the week, feeling like it's not as good as it could be, focused only getting stuff done not on the enjoyment of it.

Burnout Buster - Energy: It's not enough merely to complete the tasks on your list, it's also important to find or rediscover the joy in what you do. Are there ways you could timetable moments of calm to ponder the how not just the what? A walk outside, a different venue for a meeting, new people to share ideas with, more partnerships?

33. You are relying on 'quick fixes'. Self-medication

You can't work too hard, for too long, ignoring your health, without the use of some kind of sticking plaster or 'quick fix'.

It is possible to manage an unusually busy time through good eating, meditation and yoga, but even then, there's a limit to how long you can carry on at the same pace. For most mortals we end up 'self-medicating' using alcohol, food, sugar, over-spending, gambling or playing mind-numbing games on the computer. We are looking for something to keep us going, or keep us sane, but by using a quick fix, we're storing up other problems.

Real Stories: Daksha is a full-time consultant, travelling up and down the country delivering great quality to her customers. She's also set up her own business and at weekends she is a full time 24 hour carer for her mother who is very ill. Wow, a prime candidate for burnout eh? Yet every time I see her she's bright and positive and rarely gets ill. So, what's her secret? The key thing is her mantra that self-care is non-negotiable. She really cannot have the life she currently has of she was using 'quick fixes' like junk food, caffeine or sugar. Medium to long term she would go 'pop'. So, yoga, meditation, quiet time, coaching to off-load the pressure and good nutrition is essential to Daksha's week. She stays aware of how she's feeling and responds healthily if something starts to feel off balance.

I do a lot of those things too because I've learned the hard way that it's the best way. I have to admit I take my eye off the ball from time to time and get reminded of my own teachings by paying the consequences then getting back on it!

Burnout Buster - Energy: Notice what choices you're making, if it's something that is going to help short term you might decide it's worth it. The key is to stay conscious of those choices and know that when you're relying on them long term, you're going to need a more sustainable way to cope.

If you're experiencing difficult circumstances that are going to continue, you can meditate all you like, but if you're driving two hours a day to a job you hate, single-handedly doing the tasks of 4 people or being repeatedly bullied, sooner or later you might choose to face up to the real problem. There comes a point when you have to stop masking the problem with quick fixes and make a brave (even scary) but necessary change for the future. You'll thank yourself in the end, and your health and happiness will flourish as a result. You really are worth it.

An Executive Summary

Some of the riskiest burnout behaviours seem to be the ones I see most often!

I place them here as a reminder and a warning to us all, myself included:

- **I'm invincible!** You think you are right. And you think you're invincible. You think because you've managed something once, you can carry on pushing your luck. You need a way to conduct an honest reality check. Do you want to be right or do you want to be healthy?

- **You don't listen.** You take a big risk when you stop listening to the people who have your best interests at heart, they can see the things you are ignoring. Listen to them.

- **You miss the clues.** Ignoring the little (or massive) red flags that are telling us to find balance. Stop ignoring them, they WILL get bigger. Do something different.

- **You focus on the wrong things.** My contributors included here and the many others who have informed my work over the years, have all said this: You look back and realise the stuff you were focused on and stressed about really wasn't so important, even though it felt like it at the time, it's an illusion. There are more important things and the most important one is your health. At least step back and have a look.

- **You go on too long.** Taking a break earlier means you recover faster. The longer you pretend it's not a problem, the longer and harder your recovery.

- **You stop doing the good stuff.** Don't underestimate the little things; walking the dog, going for a swim, reading a book for pleasure, a weekend away. If you pepper your life with pleasures, it really stops the build-up and keeps you alert to the flags.

- **You're in disaster mode.** Everyone needs a wellbeing strategy. If you often give more than you have in your tank, you really have to have a wellness plan or make plans for your burnout. I'd really rather you plan for wellbeing than disaster.

If you're also an employer or manager or in any way have responsibility for the welfare of those around you, consider their burnout risk and whether they are falling in to any of the behaviours mentioned here.

Whilst running training courses on stress reduction and resilience staff have told me "My boss tells me to take lunch and go home on time, but he doesn't, so I guess he would think if I'm as committed to the job as he is, I'll put more hours in."

You need to realise that you are a role model whether you like it or not. If you aren't going home on time, having a lunch break or generally looking after yourself, the unwritten message is that you expect the same from your staff – even if you tell them the opposite. Just like children, we more often take our cues from what we see, not what we're told.

What do your people need and what kind of culture does your team, family or organisation have; does it foster wellbeing or burnout?

Look out for those Red Flags and don't then drive on regardless. Drive with caution and don't overtake your own health.

What's next? And free stuff!

If you're conscious of the drivers that can send you out of balance, notice your habits, heed your Little Red Flags before they become big ones and have some ongoing maintenance habits to keep your tank topped up, you're in the best position to avoid burnout.

It's important also to keep an eye on the bigger picture. You can manage your stress, workload and wellbeing all you like, but if you're in an impossible situation or one that makes you consistently unhappy, you can't sustain wellness. Consider what big picture things need to change, not just how you're tolerating or managing the situation.

If you allow yourself the joy of noticing what you achieve each day, celebrating your skills, acknowledging even the little wins, you can feel good any time of the day because it's all in your hands.

There is so much more work needed to raise awareness of why we need the techniques and remedies I had written about. Because sorting out a disaster is much sexier than preventing it happening. Take emergency services for example; Most people get excited if a fire engine arrives at their workplace, reacting to an emergency. They really don't respond with the same excitement if it's the health and safety team popping in to talk about preventative measures.

Emergencies are so much more galvanizing than prevention and maintenance. So, we pootle along thinking we can skip meals, say 'yes' all the time, cram our diaries, ignore our immune systems, sleep badly, accrue leave days and regularly cancel social events without consequences to our health, happiness and effectiveness. There are so many ways in which we are DIS-couraged from paying attention to our health and wellbeing. Cuts in budgets, increases in workloads, tension in teams, adverts for quick fixes all mean we need to keep reminding each other to be well.

This book is a 'wake-up call'! Sign up for my Monday Motivational Message and we'll keep the message going. We're all worth it!

This little book uses the format of my C.A.R.E. Model to explain wellbeing. Have a look for my C.A.R.E. Model book to learn more about how this self-care model can improve every aspect of your wellbeing including your team and organisation.

Further Resources

Here are some completely free resources to keep your tank topped up:

A boost by email every Monday morning to help you start your week positively. If you haven't already, sign up for my Monday Motivational Message on the website: www.pamburrows.com

Check your risk with the Burnout Buster Quiz! www.pamburrows/getquiz

Check out my channel on www.YouTube.com/c/pamburrowspeoplebooster for lots of videos and audios for reducing stress and building confidence and resilience.

Install my free app for apple https://itunes.apple.com/gb/app/peoplebooster/id1075485531?mt=8

or android https://play.google.com/store/apps/details?id=com.goodbarber.peoplebooster

and get all my resources in one place. It's a kind of library of all my online resources and platforms.

Look for The CARE Model book on Facebook and Amazon in 2019

And if you'd like to talk about sustainable well-being strategies for your organisation, a keynote at your next conference or a Booster Workshop for your team, email me at pam@pamburrows.com.

Please take care of yourself. There's only one you and you are precious.
Much love,
Pam x

Printed in Great Britain
by Amazon